DON'T GET OUT OF BED YET

10 Easy Exercises to Relieve Back, Hip, and Knee Pain

Peggy Cappy

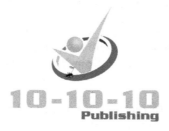

10-10-10
Publishing

DON'T GET OUT OF BED YET: 10 Easy Exercises to Relieve Back, Hip and Knee Pain
www.DontGetOutOfBedYet.com
Copyright © 2023 Peggy Cappy
Photography: Gary Gold

Paperback ISBN: 979-8-865343-89-9

Publisher
10-10-10 Publishing
Markham, ON Canada

Printed in Canada and the United States of America

*To all my yoga students past and present,
you have been my inspiration and reward.*

Table of Contents

Acknowledgments

"You have to do it by yourself, and you can't do it alone," my good friend Martin Rutte always reminds me.

Every author will tell you that statement is totally true. Writing a book is a labor of love, involving many.

My gratitude always starts with my students, past and present. They are forever in my heart and mind. Their dedication to yoga, better health, and peace of mind (and frankly, to me) is something I hold dear. I do this work for them.

The team at WGBH has been by my side for over two decades. It does not seem possible that it was 2001 when I walked into an office at WGBH in Boston and met the creative force of nature, Laurie Donnelly. She has been my great partner in promoting my message to a wide audience that yoga can change your life. And thank you, David Berstein, for that first conversation that opened the door to the success of "yoga for the rest of us"; my goodness, what long legs it has had. To Scott Sauer of Albany's WMHT, and VP of PBS Distribution, pledge master extraordinaire, thank you for knowing this book would be a great combo as we created the bonus gifts for the *5-Minute Yoga Fix*. Also, I would like to thank the extended family of co-workers at WGBH and PBS for all their support and hard work over the years.

To my photographer for this project, Gary Gold, all I can say is I really like how you make me look. Thank you for taking a cover shot that captures the joy that yoga brings me every day, as well as all the photos of me illustrating the exercises so that you, the reader, would have a visual reference to go by.

Warm thanks to Martin Rutte, who not only was the first person to welcome me into the Transformational Leadership Council but also became a writing buddy in our Get Your Book Done club, as he worked on the sequel to his book *Project Heaven of Earth*, called *Paradise Found*. A huge thank you to the rest of our group: Kian Gohar, co-author of *Competing in the New World of Work*; Donna Steinhorn and Cherie Clark, whose amazing books are yet to be published; and sadly, Elisabeth Misner, who passed on just a month before her book *Called Out of the Church* was published. Through it all, we laughed and loved and held the light for each other. How lucky I am. A thank you as well to Gail Woodard, whose online writing group gave me a gentle, regular time to write.

"WOW" is all I can say about Raymond Aaron. His inspirational 10-10-10 writing program gave me the structure and support to put words on the page and see this book come to life. A big thank you to him also for penning the foreword. And to Raymond's team, including my wonderful book architect Naval Kumar, Liz Ventrella, Lisa Browning, Waqas, and others for the guidance, editing, and design help to bring my vision to a completed book. You are all superb and I could not have done this without you. A special additional thank you to Raymond's daughter, Emma Aaron, who at the age of 15 published her book, *# Success.* Her book is the perfect example of how to become a successful author.

There are always so many people who inspire us. I have been blessed with a very, very rich life in this way. Lee Albert has been one of the most recent pivotal influences in my understanding of just how this body of ours works, and his knowledge and his generosity are amazing (*Yoga for Pain Relief* and *Live Pain-Free.*) Gratitude also to the doctors and physical therapists, and of course yoga teachers by the score, people from whom I have gained so much knowledge over the years, not only about how my own body responds to injury and aging, but also about growth and connection with spirit.

And always by my side, whenever I most need her, is my wonderful, forever friend Debra Boudrieau. My absolute gratitude and love to you for your big-hearted spirit and your amazing knowledge of all things needed, whether by me or the entire state of Vermont!

Acknowledgements always end with family; I think because we just naturally save the best for last. To my sister, Linda Orr, who is not only one of my best friends but my devoted assistant in this work, I love you. My children Leela and Zennet, and their partners Eddie and Pauline, who all live life so fully and continue to fill my heart with appreciation and love. To my granddaughters Isabelle and Elliana, beautiful young women of grace and power, and my grandsons Erol and Tau, fierce and amazing young spirit warriors.

And to my love, Alan, for every day.

Foreword

When Peggy Cappy told me about her newest approach to yoga, the first thing I said was, "Go write the book. People need this now."

And she did. Because Peggy believes in yoga and its restorative healing powers more than anyone I have ever met. Peggy has devoted her life to yoga. She knows her stuff. She has been practicing and teaching yoga for more than 50 years, and is the bestselling star of the public television series *Yoga for the Rest of Us*.

Peggy has always taken a very innovative approach to yoga. Her first video in the PBS series was based on her Gentle Stretch class (average age 74) which was really yoga in disguise using chairs. This book is equally inventive. And easy. Easier than any other yoga approach Peggy has ever undertaken.

This yoga is done in bed. Before your feet hit the floor. Ten short, easy exercises to do right after you wake up. These sequences – pick one or two or three (or get really addicted to how great they make you feel and do all ten) – will stretch out the tight places in your legs, hips, and back and will transform your body. If you miss a morning, do these exercises when you are back in bed at the end of the day before sleep, to release tension, and aches and pains.

Do yourself and your body a big favor and gift yourself this book, and Peggy's incredible wisdom. You will be very glad you did.

Raymond Aaron
New York Times **Bestselling Author**

A Personal Note

"WHACK!"

That terrible sound of a bird flying into my window jolted me out of my blissful morning reverie. I love sitting in front of the huge wall of windows, looking out over the field and lake that is my front yard, to the mountain beyond. The large windows bring the beautiful, serene view to me and connect me to nature through all the seasons, and I begin my day in joy and peace.

Hearing that crash, though, caused me to jump. I looked on the deck below the window and found a small yellow bird, an American Goldfinch. It was stunned and not moving. Then I saw it blink. I was relieved it was still alive. I silently whispered a prayer and hoped the bird would recover; indeed, when I looked later, the bird was gone.

Not long after, while at my car dealership, I heard that terrible "whack" again. It was a brilliantly sunny, autumn day when I stopped to check on an auto part I had ordered. When I learned it would take another day, I headed back down the hall and outside through a large, wide open, sliding door. I kept moving and hit that solid plate glass window so hard. "Smack!" I slammed backwards and fell hard to the floor. My very first thought was a flash of knowing exactly how that little bird must have felt—confused and dazed.

Before I could assess what had happened and how I was feeling, one of the salesmen came over and said, "Oh! Are you OK?"

"I just need a moment to collect myself." My brain must have been taking an inventory and fortunately found no broken bones or obvious injury.

Obviously distressed to find a woman on the floor, he said, "The cleaning crew just removed the taped stickers that were on the glass." I recommended that he now put something in front of the glass so that no one else would make the mistake I made. He immediately rolled a tire in front of the glass (where it remains to this day.)

Fortunately, my sister was waiting for me in the car outside. I told her what happened. I was shaken but grateful that I was not injured. I knew it could have been bad with the force of that collision; my body-in-motion being stopped instantly by the plate glass. I thought at the time that I was not seriously injured because I could walk away.

Weeks later, I began having trouble with pain in my left hip, but I did not connect my pain to the accident. Over the next few weeks, the hip pain got worse. I stopped being able to sit in my favorite cross-legged position for meditation. Then I stopped my daily walks. I was still able to do yoga daily, but it seemed like the more I moved, the more it hurt. I was stuck in an unfamiliar place.

I have been teaching yoga since the 1970s, and over the last two decades, I have made eleven yoga video programs for public television. I know yoga helps relieve pain, often more quickly than anything else. My courses are called "Yoga for the Rest of Us" and "Easy Yoga for...," to emphasize just how easy and simple yoga can be. The series is for busy, working folks who do not have hours a day to devote to a yoga practice; or, for those who are injured and need a gentle approach to get the body back in action.

I want my teaching to help everyone learn how simple and helpful yoga can be. I know that what benefits me also helps my students and those new to yoga.

Pain is often the motivator for someone to begin a yoga class or to seek private instruction. Pain can be a constant, insistent voice and an annoyance that drives a person to seek relief.

Yoga teacher Olga Kabel says, "Pain might reflect the body part's desire to protect the student and prevent further damage, or to bring attention to the area that needs to be cared for. Either way, looking at painful areas as protectors rather than troublemakers might help students feel more compassion and understanding toward those parts."

For me, my pain was like a flashing neon sign: "Pay Attention Here!" Not understanding yet where the pain came from, I wondered if I might need a hip replacement. The X-ray of my hip revealed good news. My hip looked "normal for a woman my age." No hip replacement needed. Physical therapy was recommended.

When I met my physical therapist, Jane, she asked me if I had fallen or been in an accident. I immediately remembered slamming into the plate glass and recoiling from the impact. I could see it happening again, this time in my mind, and really felt how much my hip was impacted by the blow. It was almost as if my connective tissue held me tight during the catastrophe, but then it forgot to let me go.

Jane was a gem. She focused on releasing the tight connective tissue of my hip and thigh. After each visit, the pain in my hip became less intense. I felt her work undoing places of tightly held tension.

I was also motivated to explore stretching, exercises, and yoga poses that might maintain my relief. The good news: I discovered that stretching in bed was a great way to stretch tight muscles as well as a proactive way to start the day!

Even with the pain long gone, I continue to do daily stretches in bed. Stretching is a great way to begin the day. I teach the same movement sequences to my yoga students. They all exclaim how good the "floor" work is (because, of course, they do the exercises on their yoga mats rather than in bed. You can, too, if you prefer.).

As I think back to my hip problem caused by the accident, I now see the good that came of it, strange enough to say. In my experimentation to figure out what I could do to relieve the pain, I came up with these powerful movement sequences for the hips, legs, and back. There is also a simple move for releasing neck tension and headaches, and a bonus pose to relieve sciatica.

I continue to use these exercises as a start to my day to help maintain a healthy, supple, happy body. I want that for you too. Join me now.

Introduction

Thank you for choosing this book. I know there are a wealth of yoga lessons available, and I am thrilled you have chosen mine.

This was written with you in mind, someone who is way too busy to stop and take a yoga class.

I want to show you how you can make time for stretching, in just a few minutes a day, before you get out of bed, or possibly when you return to bed before sleep.

Each of the lessons takes only a minute or two. You can do them in 5-minute sequences. They are the result of years of my yoga practice and teaching.

You do not need months of practice to benefit from the lessons here. You need just a few minutes a day and, in very short order, you will feel the difference that these exercises make to your well-being.

Before you begin, read this section.

Getting Started

- Stretching Like a Dog or Cat
- What? Yoga Stretches in Bed?
- Imbalances in Back, Hips, Knees and What that Costs You
- How to Get the Most from These Exercises
- You Decide
- The Pain-Free Way: 60-80% vs 100% Effort

Watch a dog or cat right when they awaken, whether from a full night's sleep or even just a nap. What do they do?

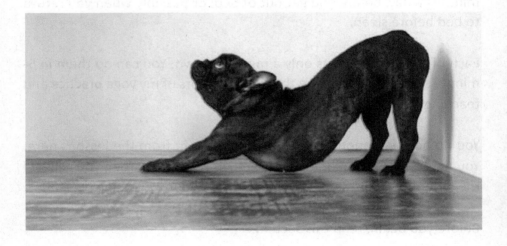

They stretch. They stretch their entire spine and all four legs. It looks like it feels so good. Your dog or cat acts out of instinct for what its body needs. Our furry critters do not need to "undo" the effects of sitting all day like most of us do, so it does not take them long to stretch after being curled up for a while.

What if you did the same, just like a dog or cat? Begin stretching immediately after awakening...before you get up and get on the move.

I will show you 10 "feel-good stretches" and movement sequences that you can do from bed. Discover how easy it is to wake up your body and create a great start to the day.

What stops you from exercising if you are not one to do it? Are you unsure of what to do? If so, you are holding terrific instructions to start you on your way.

Or do you plan to work out sometime later in the day...and find that you seldom get around to it? Maybe, for you, life gets busy the moment your feet touch the ground. If so, stretch before you begin your busy day, or at last resort, when you climb back into bed for sleep.

Here is how:

When you awaken, do this quick stretch: Bring your arms over your head and press your heels away from you. Stretch your entire body, reaching your hands and arms overhead and your legs and feet as far as you can in the other direction. Then if you need to, throw the bed covers back, make a quick trip to the bathroom, return to bed, and lie down on your back to stretch a bit more.

Back in bed, stretch more on the right side of your body, then switch and stretch the left side. One arm and leg as far as you can, then the opposite side. Next, stretch both sides equally again. After stretching like that, relax your whole body. There. Your dog/cat stretch is complete.

Exercise 1 is no more complicated than that. It will do wonders for your feet and ankles, which affect your balance and your mobility, and it takes only a minute. Who ordinarily thinks about ankle exercise?

All the following poses and exercises are easy to do and easy to learn. They will tone and balance the muscles of your front, back, and sides. The repetitive sequences will lubricate your joints, especially your hips and lower back. The movement increases oxygen and blood flow to your muscles and tissues. Best of all, you will begin the day truly renewed.

Without stretching, many of your muscles may be stuck in an out-of-balance condition, most likely from sitting too long at your desk, or in front of the computer or TV. Or maybe you suffer from neck strain from repeatedly moving your head and neck too far forward over your torso when you use your phone to text, read, or play games.

Many aches and pains throughout the body originate from muscle imbalance—some muscles get tight with tension, while others become weak from being repeatedly overstretched. If you live with muscle imbalance month after month and year after year, an unfortunate condition sets in and your body starts to wear out unevenly. This leads to back, hip, or knee problems...Like the tires on a car wear unevenly when the front end is out of alignment.

If you have chronic back pain, knee, hip, or foot pain, it is likely that your hip muscles are out of alignment, resulting in strain and pain.

The good news is that the imbalances are not difficult to fix, using the simple stretches I show you here. They work, and they will work for you, even if you have let the condition persist for so long that you can hardly remember living pain-free. I will literally show you how to get back the feeling of a younger, pain-free body.

Think back to your high school physical science class; you may remember that it is the bones of the body that create our structure and give us our form. The bones connect to each other through joints. Your bones cannot move on their own. It is the muscles in your body that move your bones. And all muscles that move your bones are paired. To move a bone, one muscle contracts while another gets pulled long.

As you move through the day, many movements you make are repetitive ones. For example, your ankle flexes with every step you take. Step after step, you lead with your heel. Seldom do you stretch the top of your foot and lead with your toe. That would be called a "dance walk." It would look and feel weird to go around that way unless you were on the stage.

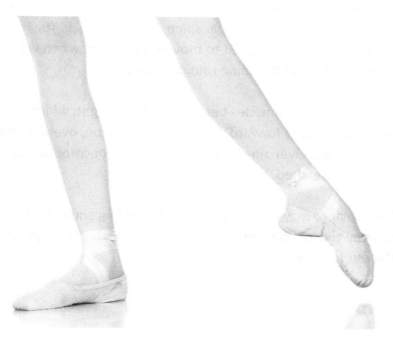

As a result, the muscles on the tops of your feet may become shorter and tighter. That can result in painful conditions like plantar fasciitis or arthritis. I know this from experience because of pain I had in my left big toe. When the pain first developed, I thought there was nothing I could do about it, except live with it. I figured the arthritis was a result of an injury many decades ago, way back when I was in fifth grade. I stumbled during a "potato sack" relay race and broke my big toe. The arthritis, decades later, was a result of that long-ago event.

Then I learned that I could get rid of the pain simply by stretching the top of my foot. With a gentle foot stretch held for two minutes, all the pain went away! Even better, the arthritis pain never came back. Why? Because I regularly add a "muscle-balancing" foot stretch to my daily stretches.

Think about how often, and how long, you sit during a day. Your body is not designed for long periods of sitting in a chair, especially when sitting without good support for the lumbar spine, the lower back. The natural curve in the low back is designed to move inward; yet, when we sit in most chairs, that part of the spine rounds outward.

If you slump, your chest muscles become short and tight, which causes your shoulders to round forward. Your back rounds too, overstretching your back muscles. Over time, the back muscles become weak and chronically overstretched.

A muscle imbalance may not be noticeable as a young adult. But decade after decade, those patterns register and often become painfully obvious in our later years.

When your spine stays in a C-shape, your lower back feels the pinch of lots of pressure, ultimately causing lower back pain. Sitting for long periods continues the imbalance in your hips. The muscles in your front groin contract, tighten, and pull on your pelvis as well. Over and over, throughout your body, the same muscles contract while the opposing muscles are pulled long. The muscles that are pulled long become over-stretched, weak, and tight. One muscle is contracted and tight; the other is over-stretched and tight.

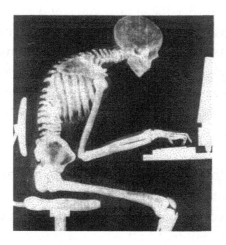

There is a remedy for both. If contracted and tight, you put the muscle in a slack position and hold the pose for a minute or two to re-set it. You also need to stretch that muscle. Conversely, muscles that have repeatedly been over-stretched need to be strengthened, not stretched, to come into balance. You will find a good and simple way to strengthen your back muscles in Exercise 5.

Out-of-balance muscles pull the bones out of alignment. The muscles become painful, and the joints get repeatedly strained, resulting in joint pain, or arthritis or bursitis. You may develop a limited range of motion in the joint as well.

The next time that you sit at your desk, or on your couch, notice if your head juts forward of your chest. This head-forward position puts strain on your neck and shoulder muscles. Unsupported or strained posture can make the muscles of your neck and back hurt, your shoulders ache, or give you a headache by the end of the day.

If you cannot picture your usual posture, get a friend or family member to take a photo of you when you are sitting down and not trying to hold yourself in good posture. Look at how you stand without trying to stand up straight. And observe your colleagues, friends, and neighbors.

To undo the effects of bad sitting or poor standing posture, and to rebalance the muscles in your body, start the day stretched and strong. This book will help you learn how to stretch. Your dilemma may simply be how to fit stretching exercises into a busy life when it feels like you have no time to spare.

One way is simply to decide to do a few stretching exercises every day. Make an agreement with yourself to do daily exercises in bed for one week. Notice how you feel after several consecutive days. If you do the exercises daily, you will feel better and you will not mind taking the couple minutes to start your day stronger.

Repeat the next week, adding a new or additional exercise to the mix.

Experts say it takes about 30 days to instill a new habit. If you want to feel better, give yourself at least 10 minutes of stretching for 30 days. If you think that you do not have a couple of minutes to spare once you open your eyes, then set your alarm for ten minutes earlier than your usual time for getting up. The benefits will outweigh the missed ten minutes of sleep; I promise. You will have to try this to know for yourself.

The first set of exercises starts in the next chapter. They take only one or two minutes. Exercise 1 is the place to begin. Over time, try each of the 10 stretching-in-bed exercises. See which ones work best for you and bring needed relief. The entire set of reclining exercises in this book may take you 30 minutes or more. If 30 minutes seems too long to commit to every day, go ahead and choose the exercises that feel most beneficial, always starting with your feet. You may wish to do the whole set of exercises on a day off from work or when you have more time in the morning.

If all else fails, take your 10 minutes when you are back in bed at the end of the day. Doing an exercise or two at the end of the day will help relax your body for a good night's sleep.

Here is a surprise: 10 minutes out of your day is only 1% of your waking time. You can afford to spend 10 minutes, or 1% of your time, on the self-care of stretching.

Oh, and one other important thing to help you: Many people follow the dictum: "No pain, no gain." That is **not** the case here. My exercises are no pain, all gain.

Instead of doing each set of movements at 100% capacity, make your range of movement only about 60–80% of your maximum to bring a greater sense of ease to the exercises.

I warn you: It will be difficult to remember not to give it "your all." If/when you notice that you are stretching to your max, back off a little. You will find greater comfort and ease, and your stretch will be more effective and easier to hold than when done at 100% capacity.

Why? Because at 60–80% of your range of movement, you are stretching the belly of the muscle. At 100%, you put tension and strain on the tendons, the places where the muscles attach to the bones. You want these exercises to benefit the muscles, not strain the tendons. And believe me, it is going to feel better to do less than your maximum.

Turn the page to see the perfect way to begin. I promise you that your gain will be greater than the loss of a couple minutes of your time.

Chapter 1

Exercise 1 – Rejuvenate Stiff Ankles for Better Balance and Mobility

Begin with a simple and easy-to-learn routine for your feet and ankles.

My experience teaching yoga for many decades has revealed that by regularly exercising your feet and ankles, you will:

- **Increase circulation** to your feet (which is especially important for people whose circulation to the extremities is compromised).
- **Strengthen the muscles.** (Did you know that the muscles in your hands and feet comprise more than half of all the muscles in your body?)
- **Create more flexibility** in the ankle joints (making you less likely to shuffle in your advanced years).
- **Experience more resiliency** and gain the ability to recover from a misstep.
- **Improve your balance** when all your weight is on one leg; you will have the support you need to make fine adjustments in the supporting foot and ankle.

These exercises for your feet and ankles are easy to learn. Do them daily. They are a great way to start your day.

Exercise 1: Feet, Toes, Ankles

1. Heel Press
2. Alternate Feet with Point and Flex
3. Circle Feet Same Direction, Reverse
4. Circle Feet Towards One Another, Reverse

1. Heel Press

Your simple starting position is called Reclining Mountain Pose.

Mountain Pose is a standing pose. But here we use it when supine, on our backs. It is easy.

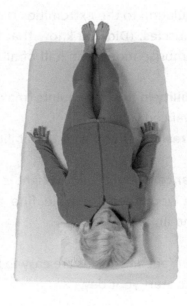

- Straighten your legs and lift your toes to the ceiling.
- Bring your arms down to your sides, palms down.
- Rotate your palms to face up, thumbs pointing outward.
- Tuck your chin in slightly towards your chest.
- Still your movement and feel yourself breathing.
- Breathe in deeper...and breathe out slower.

By paying attention to your breathing while in this simple, deliberate position, you take your awareness away from thoughts and towards an immediate awareness of your body.

The benefit? Full attention to any part of your body, or to your breath, redirects your brain and your thoughts. It inhibits worrying or over-thinking a situation or problem. It may allow you to experience inner stillness and inner silence.

Ultimately, with practice, you learn to calm yourself in any stressful moment, by slowing down your breathing, extending the exhalation to double the length of the inhalation, and watching each breath come in and go out.

Now, to "wake up" your feet:

- Slowly and gently press your heels away from your body while pulling your toes towards you. Spread your toes wide if you can.

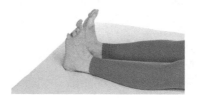

- Hold this position for one slow, full breath.
- Slowly point your toes, extending your ankles.

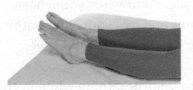

- Pull your toes back again, spread the toes, and press through your heels.
- Continue to slowly point your toes; flex your toes and ankles 5 or more times.
- Rest briefly. Relax your feet and legs. Let your feet flop out to the sides instead of returning to Reclining Mountain Pose.

2. Alternate Feet with Point and Flex

- Pull your right toes back and press your heel forward while you point your left toes and extend that foot.

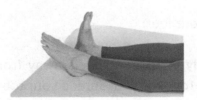

- Continue alternating the movement of the feet, 5 or more times.
- Relax and rest.

3. Circle Feet Together, Same Direction

Add these movements to strengthen the muscles around your ankles and to increase the flexibility of your ankle joints. With your feet together, inner edges touching:

- Circle your toes and feet to the left and around in a circle.

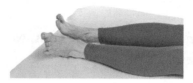

- Complete 5, or more, foot circles.
- Circle the feet together in the other direction.
- Relax your feet and rest for a moment, sensing how your ankles feel.

4. Circle Feet Towards One Another

- Separate your feet to be wider than hip-width apart.
- Slowly circle your feet towards each other and around.

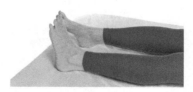

- Complete 5 or more circles.

- Change the direction of the foot circles to the other direction.

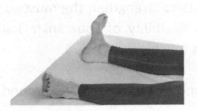

Relax and feel the effects.

Take a deep breath in and a slow breath out. Notice the sensation in your toes...feet...ankles...calves.

How would you describe those sensations in one or two words?

Whisper "Hurray!" to celebrate completing the first exercise.

Then lightly smile and enjoy "not doing anything" for three breaths.

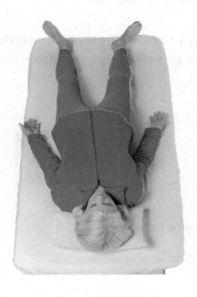

You have finished Exercise 1. Hasn't it been easy?

Want to know how to make this short exercise a new mini habit?

Decide to do it daily. And once done, do celebrate your completion each time with a quiet but enthusiastic response: "Hooray!" or "Woohoo!"

Done on a regular basis, you will strengthen the muscles of your feet and ankles, increase the circulation in your feet, and make your ankle joints supple and flexible. In time, your balance will be steadier and your feet "happier."

That is what happened for Cherie, who has done the Exercise 1 footwork daily for months. She says, "My left ankle no longer swells and both ankles are stronger. An additional success is that my balance is definitely better."

Move on to the next chapter to begin your legwork. I promise the next exercise section will feel as good or better, for your legs and hips.

Chapter 2

Exercise 2: Preliminary Hip Stretch

While lying on your back in Reclining Mountain Pose:

1. Knee to Chest
2. Crossed Knee Pull

If you are comfortable without a pillow under your head, do without.

If your neck muscles are tight and your chin juts up to the ceiling without a pillow, the lift of a pillow will bring your nose and chin into the same plane. It may simply feel more comfortable to lie down with a pillow under your head.

1. Knee to your chest, right leg:

- Bend your right knee and pull your knee into your chest.
- As you hold your right knee, keep your right foot soft and relaxed.
- Your left leg remains straight. Press through your left heel.

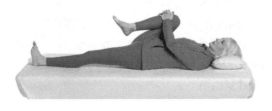

By flexing the ankle of your straight leg, you engage the muscles of the entire leg. That foot and leg will feel different from the foot and leg that remains relaxed. You may find that the foot of your bent knee automatically flexes when the straight leg does, so work to keep the foot of the bent knee relaxed.

Feel the opposition: Your right knee is being pulled in one direction while your left heel presses in the opposite direction.

- Hold your right knee for 5 slow breaths in and out. This pose relaxes muscles in your hips. The pressure of thigh against abdomen stimulates your lower digestive system. Specifically, the right knee into the chest gently compresses the ascending colon.
- Release your hold and straighten your right leg. Rest your right leg next to your left and notice any difference in sensation between right and left legs.

Left knee to your chest:

- Bend your left knee and pull it into your chest.
- Hold for 5 breaths. On this side, the left thigh gently compresses the descending colon.
- Release your left leg and stretch it out next to your right leg. Relax your entire body.
- Take a deep breath in, and a long, slow breath out.

This easy position of "holding your knee into your chest" puts the psoas muscle into a slack position, causing that muscle to release tension. The psoas muscle is located deep in your hip area on each side; it connects your upper body to your lower half. A hold in this position will often ease back pain and strain.

Do you feel more ease in your hip joints?

2. Crossed Knee Pull

This is a very powerful exercise to gently stretch the outer hip and relieve tension in the hip muscles.

- Bend both knees and place the feet on the bed with knees and feet touching.
- Cross the right leg over the left.
- Clasp the right knee and gently pull it towards you.

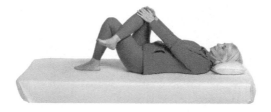

- Hold here, or to deepen the stretch, lift your left foot off the bed.

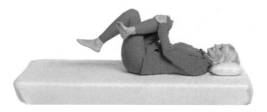

- Hold for a minimum of one minute.
- Then uncross the legs and repeat on the other side.

This completes Exercise 2. Do you feel more freedom in your hip joints?

In the next chapter, you will move both legs symmetrically, at the same time, into a few reclining yoga poses. Turn to the next chapter and give it a try.

Chapter 3

Exercise 3: Hips and Lower Back: Both Legs, Moving Together

This movement sequence helps to realign and stretch the spine and may relieve lower back pain. The combined poses improve the flexibility of the hips. The final resting position lowers the heart rate; the entire sequence helps ease stress and anxiety.

1. Knees to Chest
2. Bound Angle Pose (*Baddha-Konasana*)
3. Happy Baby Pose (*Ananda Balasana*)
4. Reverse Flow

1. Knees to Chest

- Bring both knees into your chest, with a hand on each knee and feet relaxed. Draw your chin towards your chest.

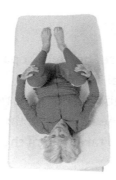

- Hold for at least 3 breaths, and up to 10 breaths to increase the benefits of the pose.
- This first pose in this sequence is also called "wind-relieving pose," as the legs squeeze out gas trapped in the intestines, relieving flatulence, which is often a source of abdominal discomfort.

2. Bound Angle Pose

- Bring the bottoms of your feet together as you separate your knees.

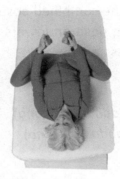

- Move your knees wide to the sides.
- Use your hands on your feet, ankles, or lower legs to draw your feet closer to your chest while knees stay wide apart.
- Hold the position; breathe a minimum of three breaths.

3. Happy Baby Pose

- From Bound-Angle Pose, begin to separate your feet and lift each foot up towards the ceiling.
- Place your right foot above your bent right knee and your left foot above your left bent knee, hands to the back of your knees.
- If flexible, reach up and take hold of the outer edges of your legs or feet.

- Draw your knees as close to your sides as possible.

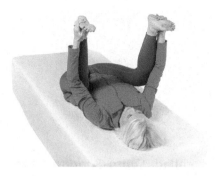

My granddaughter Isabelle was only six months old when, much to my surprise, she spontaneously performed this pose—she was on her back during a diaper change. A look of delight registered on her face as she grabbed each foot, and she laughed out loud.

This is a pose that you, too, most likely did when you were just a baby. While trying out this pose, imagine yourself as a baby, innocently doing the pose just because you can!

4. Reverse Flow

- Bring your feet back together with your knees outward, returning to Bound Angle Pose.
- Gently pull your feet towards you.
- Take a slow breath in and out.
- Next, keep your knees wide with feet together, and lower your feet to the bed.

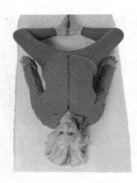

This yoga pose is called *Supta-Baddha-Konasana* in Sanskrit and translates to "Reclining Bound-Angle Pose." This pose stretches the inner thigh and groin muscles, and when held, it helps relieve symptoms of stress and anxiety.

- Hold the position while slowly breathing in and out, for up to a minute.
- Then bring your knees together and place your feet on the bed with knees bent.
- Straighten your legs and rest them a little wider than hip-width apart.

Take 3 deep breaths and relax.

There is only one pose we do in the next chapter, with a few variations. The Figure 4 pose is as close to "twisting like a pretzel" as we will get, but do not let that scare you.

Figure 4 pose puts the psoas muscle (a muscle deep in the pelvis that connects your torso to your leg) into a slack position when held, often relieving strain, pain, and backache.

16

Chapter 4

Exercise 4: A Pose Like a Pretzel
Supta-EkaPadaUtkatasana in Sanskrit

1. Figure 4 Pose, Release the Psoas
2. Variations
3. Repeat the Sequence, Other Side

The psoas muscle is a big, strong muscle that attaches to the lumbar region of the spine (lower back) and moves through the pelvis to the thigh bone, the femur. It is what helps hold your top half to the lower half of your body. When you sit for long periods of time, your psoas muscles (one on each side of the spine) often contract and remain strained.

A tight psoas muscle can cause problems ranging from chronic back pain and sciatica to functional leg length discrepancy. The Figure 4 Pose helps release a tight psoas muscle. Figure 4 Pose also tones the core muscles and stretches the outer hip and gluteus muscles, benefitting hip flexibility and joint rotation.

1. Figure 4 Pose, Release the Psoas

- Begin in Reclining Mountain Pose.
- Bend both knees and place your feet on the bed, about hip-width apart.

- Lift your right foot, keeping your knee bent, and place your right ankle against the top of your left thigh. Extend your right foot a little to the left so that you rest the bone of your right lower leg against the left thigh, rather than resting directly on the ankle joint itself.

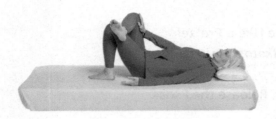

- Gently press your right knee away from you. You will likely feel this in your right hip. Feel free to stop here and hold this position.

This may be all the stretch that feels right to you in the moment. If so, maintain this position. But to go deeper into the stretch:

2. Variations

- Lift your left foot off the bed and pull your bent left knee closer to your torso.
- Thread your right hand and arm through the opening between your legs, and reach your left arm around the outside of your left thigh.
- Clasp your left shin as you pull that leg closer to you.

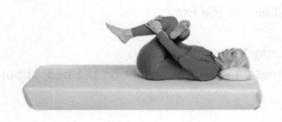

- If you cannot reach your shin, hold your thigh under your lower leg.

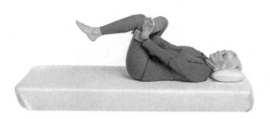

Additional Leg Variation with the Pose:

- Instead of keeping your left leg bent, straighten your left leg up to the ceiling.

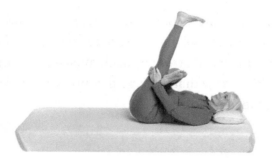

- Reach up and clasp your big toe, ankle, or lower leg.

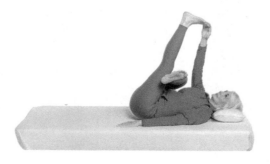

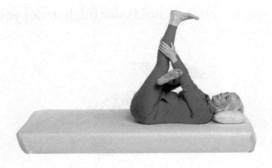

- After holding for a minute or longer, bend your knee and release that foot to the bed. Remove the right foot from the left knee and return both feet to the bed; straighten your legs and relax.

4. Repeat the Sequence, Other Side

In the next chapter, your starting position will be similar, with knees bent and feet on the bed, but we will be doing presses into the bed that will strengthen the back muscles. Stronger back muscles will improve your standing posture. Who knew that you could improve your carriage while lying on your back? Take a look.

Chapter 5

Exercise 5: Improve your Posture: Posterior Strengtheners

1. Head Press
2. Shoulder Press
3. Back of Waist Press
4. Half Bridge Pose, *Setu Bandhasana* in Sanskrit

The first part of this exercise consists of pressing various parts of your body into the bed. As simple as this seems, the pressing will strengthen your back muscles. Strong back muscles help to counter the rounding of the spine that results from long periods of sitting.

All the presses are done in the starting position for Half Bridge Pose.

During the presses, your muscles will be working without much observable change of your body from the outside.

Even better than doing this exercise on the soft surface of your bed, the half-bridge pose is more effective when done on the floor; the floor is a firmer surface to press against. If getting down to the floor (and if you can easily get back up) is not a problem for you, do give this exercise a try off the bed. In time, you may want to do all these morning exercises directly on the floor, rather than in bed.

Half Bridge Pose strengthens the neck, back, and gluteus (butt) muscles. The pose also tones the spinal muscles and nerves. This pose stimulates the abdominal organs, lungs, and thyroid. It also calms the brain, and when practiced regularly, it helps alleviate stress and mild depression.

Important: If you used a pillow under your head for the earlier exercises, take that pillow away during the Half-Bridge Pose so that your head rests directly on the bed or floor. Otherwise, you risk over-stretching your neck muscles when the buttocks and torso lift off the surface you are on.

Caution: Those who have undergone neck, back, shoulder, or spinal surgery should not do the Half-Bridge Pose. Likewise, people with a slipped disc or unregulated high blood pressure are advised to skip this pose.

However, the head and shoulder presses are beneficial for all and will strengthen the upper back muscles.

- Begin from Reclining Mountain Pose.
- Bend your knees and place your feet on the bed about hip width apart.
- Keep your arms relaxed to your sides, palms facing up.

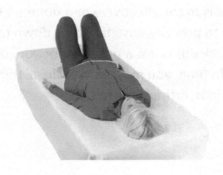

- Take a deep breath in and then a slow breath out. You will be regulating your breath with the "press and release" parts of the exercise.

1. Head Press

- Take a deep breath in, and as you begin to exhale, press the back of your head downward into the bed. Keep pressing your head downward through your entire exhalation, extending the length of the exhalation as much as you can.
- Then release and relax, taking a full breath in and out.
- Repeat the head press again, pressing the head down during the exhalation. Slow your exhalation, making the pressing last as long as possible.

2. Shoulder Press

- Continue to combine pressing on exhalation, switching now to your shoulders. After a full breath in, exhale slowly as you press your shoulders and shoulder blades down into the bed or floor.
- Repeat twice more.

3. Back of Waist Press

- Breathe in; then as you exhale, press the back of your waist into the bed/floor. Pull your navel inward towards your spine.
- Firm your abdominal area as you hold.
- Repeat twice more.

4. Half-Bridge Pose

- Begin with an inhale, and as you slowly exhale, begin pressing your shoulders down. While pressing your shoulders, simultaneously press your feet into the bed. Press into the inner edges of the feet as much as the outer edges. Lift your hips up, off the bed/floor.

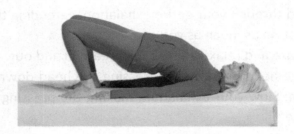

- To end the pose, lower your hips.
- Pull your knees into your chest.
- Stretch out your legs and relax.

If you choose to practice this on the floor rather than in bed, you will have a more solid base against which to press the shoulders and feet. From the floor, lifting your hips will be easier and you will be able to lift your hips higher.

While holding, keep even pressure on the bottom of the feet and do not let the knees move wider than hip-width apart as you hold the pose.

At first, you may be comfortable with holding for just a couple of breaths. Over time, you may develop the strength to hold this pose for a minute or more.

In the next chapter, you will find poses that gently turn and twist your spine. Twisting poses restore a natural range of motion to the spine and stretch the muscles of the back. They often feel good to do because they help relieve tension in the muscles that run along the spinal column. Continue to them now.

Chapter 6

Exercise 6: Twists: Realign Hips and Spine

1. Wiper Legs, Moving Twists
2. Full Twist, Knees to Chest
3. Full Twist with Top Leg Extension

Poses that twist the spine stretch the hip abductor muscles, which are the muscles on the outside of the thighs. This twist is one of the essential movements that help bring your pelvis into proper alignment.

Twists tone the spinal muscles and nerves and help to counteract slumped posture. Twists even help to release tension in your abdominal area and bring a fresh blood supply to your internal organs.

We begin with a gentle movement from side to side to initiate the changes listed above.

1. Wiper Legs, Moving Twists

- Bend your knees and place your feet on the bed, wider than hip-width apart.
- Place your arms straight out from your shoulders.

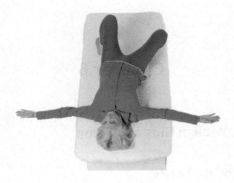

- Slowly, drop both knees down towards the right.
- Come back up to center, and then take both knees to the left.

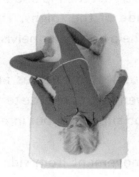

Now, add focused breathing, coordinating your breathing with the movement of the knees. Breathe out as you slowly drop your knees to the right side, and breathe in as you bring your knees back up. Drop your knees down to the left and continue.

- As you couple movement with breath, add a head movement, turning your head and neck opposite to the direction of your knees.

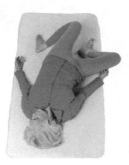

- Drop your knees to the right and turn your head to the left.
- Bring both head and knees back to center on the inhale.
- As you breathe out, bring your knees to the left as you turn your head to the right. Press both shoulders down.
- Add one more component: As you take your knees to the right, press your left foot down, and gently lift your left buttock off the bed. The left hip moves up and slightly toward the right.
- Hold for several breaths. Then repeat on the other side.

2. Full Twist, Knees to Chest

- Bring your knees into your chest.
- Place your arms out to the sides, about shoulder high.
- Slowly roll your knees over to the right while you stretch through your left arm, keeping your left shoulder on the bed.
- Place your right hand on top of your knees.
- Slowly turn your head to the left, in the direction opposite your knees.

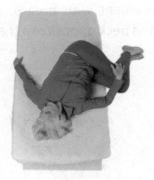

- Hold this pose for several slow breaths.
- Bring your knees back to center and hug them in.
- Place your arms back out to the sides, about shoulder high.
- Stretch through your right arm, keeping your right shoulder on the bed, and move your knees over to the left side.
- Place your left hand on top of your knees.
- Slowly turn your head to the right, in the opposite direction of your knees.
- Hold this pose while you breathe slowly.
- Bring your knees back into your chest.

3. Full Twist with Top Leg Extension

The next step is optional. It may feel good and right, or it may seem too extreme. If it causes any pain, skip it. Instead, do the twist to each side again.

- Keep both arms out to your sides, shoulder high.
- After you drop your knees to the right side, slowly straighten the top leg.
- With your right hand, grasp your knee, calf, ankle, or even the left big toe.

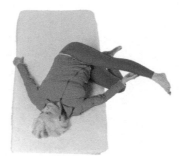

- Hold for a minute.
- Re-bend your top leg and bring your knees into your chest.
- Roll your knees over to your left and repeat as on the right side.
- Hold again for a minute.
- Re-bend your top leg and bring your knees back to your chest.
- Straighten both legs on the bed and rest for a few breaths.

Twists allow fresh oxygen and nutrients to flow to your internal organs upon release. When you pull both knees into your chest, you gently compress your organs, including the transverse colon. When you release your knees and straighten your legs on the bed, a fresh supply of blood and oxygen floods the abdominal area.

The following exercise in the next chapter will give a wonderful stretch to the back of each thigh, plus the inner and outer sides as well. Wait until you see how good your legs feel after completing these next stretches.

Chapter 7

Exercise 7: Stretch Those Legs

1. Hamstring Stretch (Back of the Thigh)
2. Inner Thigh Stretch
3. Outer Thigh and Hip Stretch
4. Leg Cycles
5. Reverse the Direction of the Cycle, Each Leg

Do you have tight hamstrings, those muscles in the backs of your thighs? What about your inner and outer thighs—are the muscles tight there as well? This next exercise will bring you ease through increased circulation.

Have a yoga strap nearby to use for these poses. If you do not have a yoga strap, you can use the belt of a bathrobe, or a towel folded lengthwise. If you are very flexible, you can extend your fingers to your toes, and take a big toe hold.

This is a longer chapter. Feel free to break your workout up into two parts: 1–3 and 4–5

1. Hamstring Stretch (Back of the Thigh)

• Begin in Reclining Mountain Pose. Take a breath in and a long breath out.

- Bend both knees and bring the bottoms of your feet to the bed.
- Bring your left knee into your chest. Place the yoga strap around the bottom of your left foot.
- Straighten the left leg up to the ceiling while holding on to the strap with both hands.

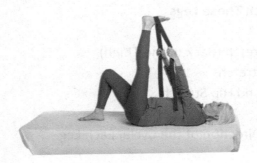

- Move your hands up the strap and clasp it so that your arms are straight, rather than keeping your elbows bent, as that will tire the muscles in your arms more quickly.

If you can easily reach your foot or ankle with your hands, you may dispense with the strap. A classic hold is to take two fingers, the index finger and the middle finger of your left hand, and place them between your left big toe and the second toe, and grasp the big toe to hold on. Proceed to straighten your left leg up to the ceiling.

- Keep your right knee bent, foot on the bed.
- Gently pull your left leg toward you.
- Hold the pose as you slow your breathing.
- Bend your knee and release the strap or your hold. Bring your foot to the bed.
- Stretch out both legs on the bed.

Notice the sensations that result after holding this pose. What is the difference in feeling between the right and left leg?

Switch Legs

- Repeat the instructions and stretch the right leg.
- After holding for an equal time as the previous leg, release your hold, set the strap aside, and stretch out both legs.
- Relax.

Notice the sensations that arise in your body as a result of finishing this pose. This is a powerful stretch.

2. Inner Thigh Stretch

- Bend both knees and place your feet on the bed.
- Pull your left knee into your chest and place your strap around the bottom of your left foot.
- Straighten your left leg up to the ceiling.

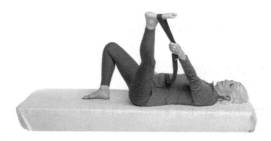

- Straighten your right leg on the bed.
- Place both sides of the strap in your left hand.
- Reach up high on the strap so that your left arm is straight.

- Place your right hand on top of your right hip bone to stabilize your pelvis and to remind yourself to keep that hip and buttock down on the bed.
- Slowly draw your left leg down to your left side.

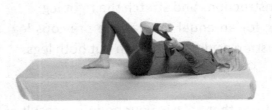

Please do not overdo the stretch to your inner thigh. See what your max is and then lift the leg to a more comfortable position. Hold the stretch to a maximum of 80% range of your flexibility.

- Hold this stretch for several deep, full breaths.
- Then lift your left leg back up to its starting place; bend your knee and remove the strap.
- Stretch out both legs on the bed.
- Relax and notice the new sensations.

Repeat these instructions for the right side.

3. Outer Thigh and Hip Stretch

We will begin with the left leg again. This time, you will be stretching your outer thigh muscles.

- Bend your knees and place both feet on the bed.
- Pull your left knee into your chest and place the strap around the bottom of your left foot.

- Straighten your left leg up to the ceiling.
- Straighten your right leg on the bed.
- Place both sides of the strap in your right hand this time and reach up high on the strap so that your right arm remains straight.
- Move your left arm out to the left side, resting it shoulder high on the bed.
- Keeping your left shoulder on the bed, draw the left leg across the body towards the right side. For now, keep both hips on the bed.

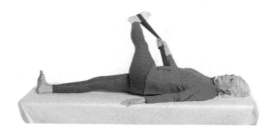

To go deeper into the stretch:

- Roll onto the right hip to draw the left leg across to the right side, without lifting your left shoulder from the bed.
- Draw the left leg as high as is comfortable, towards the right hand, out from the shoulder.
- Hold the pose while you remember to breathe deeply.

The pose gives a nice, gentle twist to the spine as well as the legs.

If you find your left shoulder lifting to enable you to stretch deeper, press that shoulder down into the bed—there is more value in the stretch when keeping both shoulders on the bed.

- Roll back to both buttocks, lifting the left leg back up to the ceiling.
- Hold on to both sides of the strap with both hands; pull your straight leg towards you, repeating the hamstring stretch.
- Hold for several breaths.
- Bend your knee, removing the strap from your foot.
- Bend your knees and place both feet on the bed.
- Lift your hips to realign your spine and hips; lower your hips back to the bed and straighten your legs to rest.

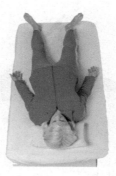

Take a moment to notice the physical effects of this twist.

Repeat the sequence for the other leg.

Once you know the three positions for the leg stretches, try doing all three on one side before switching to the other side.

Note how your legs and hips feel after this series of stretches.

4. Leg Cycles

The leg cycle lubricates the hip joints while strengthening the leg and abdominal muscles.

Cycle your left leg:

- Bend both knees and place your feet on the bed.
- Pull your left knee into your chest.

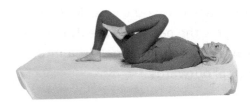

- Take a deep breath in as you slowly straighten your left leg towards the ceiling, pointing your toes. Your right leg remains bent, foot on the bed.

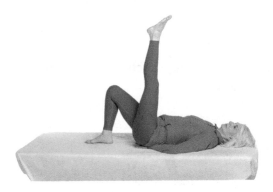

- If the back of your leg is tight, you may not be able to straighten your leg all the way.

- Place your hands on the bed, next to your hips, and slide your thumbs underneath your buttocks to support your lower back.

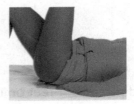

- Now flex your left ankle as you take a deep breath in. Slowly, lower your left leg towards the bed while breathing out. As you lower your leg, pull your navel and abdominal area into your body, all while pressing your heel outwards.

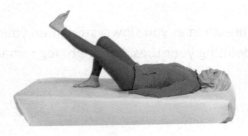

- Just before your straight leg touches the bed, re-bend the knee and pull it into your chest.

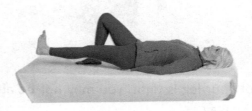

- This is one complete cycle.
- Continue the cycling movement, coordinating your breath with your leg, foot, and belly. Continue for 3 or more cycles.
- Then lower the straight leg until it touches and rests on the bed.

5. Reverse the direction of the cycle:

- Lift your left leg straight up to the ceiling, inhaling as you soften your belly and point your toes.
- Bend your knee into your chest. Relax your foot.
- As you straighten your left leg, press through your heel and extend your leg parallel to the bed. Exhale as you do this, and pull your lower abdomen into your torso with the exhalation.
- You have reversed the direction of the leg cycle.
- Complete as many cycles in this direction as you did the first direction.
- Rest for a moment and notice any differences between the sensations in your left leg and your right.

Repeat the cycle with your right leg, in both directions.

Notice how your legs and hips now feel after this series of stretches.

In this chapter, you have stretched three sides of the thighs, and lubricated your hips with the cycles.

In the next chapter, you will stretch the front of the thighs in Half-Bow Pose. Then, a unique twist will complete our active exercises. Turn the page to see what is in store.

Chapter 8

Exercise 8: Side-Lying Exercises for Back, Spine, Hips, and Thighs

1. Half-Bow Sequence
2. Rainbow Twist

Curl into a side-lying fetal position, resting on the left side. The right arm and leg are on top, and these will be the moving limbs.

Since we will do the same activity on both sides, you are welcome to start on either side once you know the sequence.

1. Half-Bow Sequence

Lie on your left side with knees and elbows bent into the body. Feel free to place a small pillow under your head. Put the pillow in place before you begin the movement.

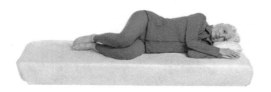

Reach your right hand to your right knee (top hand to top knee) and pull the knee into your chest.

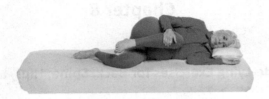

- Release your hold on the knee and straighten the top leg. As you straighten the leg, extend that leg directly in line with your torso, about two feet high above the bed.

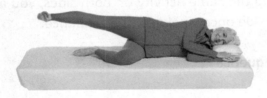

- Lift the leg a little higher; then slowly lower it all the way down to the bed. Make sure that the leg and torso are in one straight line.

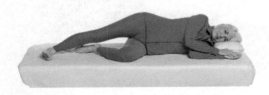

- Hold for one breath.
- Now bend the knee and reach behind you to clasp your right ankle with your right hand. (Photo 8-5) 80578

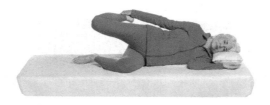

If you cannot reach your ankle, take a yoga strap or a bathrobe tie and hook it around your ankle, holding on to both ends of the strap with your right hand.

- Gently pull the foot behind you.

This will stretch the front groin as well as the front of the thigh.

- Do not allow that knee to lift. Keep your knee down near the bed for an effective stretch.

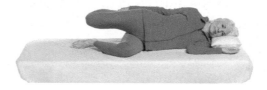

- Pull the foot and ankle back.
- Hold the pose for up to one minute, or ten slow breaths.
- If you have moved too deeply into the position, ease up without releasing the pose and continue to hold.

- Release your hold of the ankle or strap and straighten your leg out in alignment with your body once again.
- Lift the straight leg about two feet high.

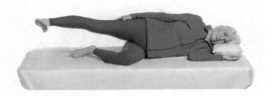

- Slowly lower the leg to the bed and hold.

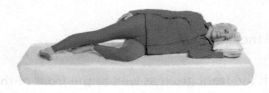

- Relax and re-bend your knee and hug it into your chest.
- Release to your starting position.

This exercise stretches the muscles in the front groin, the ones that get tight from sitting too long.

2. Rainbow Twist

- Extend your arms straight out from your heart area, resting on the bed, palms together.

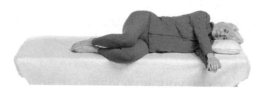

- As you slowly breathe in, begin to raise your right arm up in the air.
- Allow your eyes to follow the movement of your right hand until your hand is directly overhead

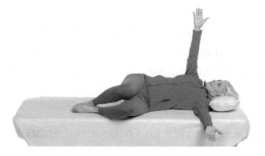

- Breathe out as you continue the arching movement until your right arm and hand rest on the bed on the other side of you.

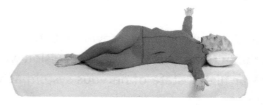

- Do not force the arm if you have shoulder limitation.

You have just carved a large arc, like a rainbow across the sky.

- Hold for a breath or two.
- Then lift your right arm up and retrace the arc back to your starting position.

Optional visualization: Use your imagination to envision rainbow colors streaming out of your fingers as you carve the arc of movement.

- Repeat the sequence again.
- Release and return to the starting position, with elbows pulled into the fetal position.

This twist is different from earlier twists we have done. Previously, we kept the shoulders on the bed and moved the hips from side to side. This time, we keep the hips stationary and move the shoulder to create the twist.

- Curl up on your other side and repeat the entire sequence on your second side.

The next chapter is a boon for relieving tight neck and shoulder muscles; the position may relax the muscles enough to help relieve an on-coming headache. Good news: The resting position is super easy to do.

This is the first time we will add eye movements to our pose. Why? Eye movements to the periphery of your range of vision work to help move us from a "fight or flight" state of nervous system activation, to "rest and digest" instead.

There is more explanation in the next chapter.

Chapter 9

Exercise 9: Pain Relief for Neck and Headache

Reclining Head Tilt

The following position of the neck and head puts the neck muscles on one side into a slack position.

- Lie down on your back.
- Place your forearm on top of your head and let your arm rest in this position.
- Tilt your head gently toward the raised upper arm.
- Hold this position, breathe slowly, and relax for two full minutes.

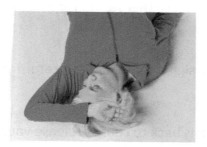

- Repeat on the other side for another two minutes.

Practice this simple pose regularly for chronic headache relief as well as to release tight muscles in your neck and shoulders. Once you have practiced this pose in bed, you can also repeat it while sitting up.

A student named Tracy benefits incredibly from this one pose. Tracy says that she often used to suffer with migraine headaches. However, now, she practices this pose daily—not just once but as much as four or five times a day—to keep tension from building in her neck and shoulders. "It has been a godsend!" she says.

There is an addition to this pose that is easy to do and consists of adding a movement for the eyes.

- When the head is tilted to the right, focus your eyes on a point in front of you.
- Slowly move your eyes to look left, opposite the direction of your head tilt.
- Gently focus on a point in your peripheral vision, as you continue to hold your head tilt.

Do not strain your gaze. Hold the focus of the eyes to the left and wait.

Your body may give you a subtle response of a sigh, yawn, or swallow during your hold. If so, use that sign to return the gaze to center, ending the fixed gaze.

If there is no subtle sign after 2 minutes, return your eyes and head to center.

- Once your head is back to center, release your arm to your side.
- Move to the second side of your neck stretch.
- Repeat the eye movement with the head tilted to the other side. When your head is tilted left, the eyes look right, and when the head is tilted right, the eyes look left.

- Hold and wait for two minutes or release the eye hold upon the subtle response from your body. Keep your head tilted for a full 2 minutes.

Engaging the eyes to the peripheral position with a hold activates the vagus nerve, part of the parasympathetic nervous system.

The vagus nerve is the longest nerve in the body; it runs from the brain stem through the eyes, ears, and tongue, to the chest, and continues down the body, connecting to all the major organs and the digestion system.

The vagus nerve has garnered much attention in relation to relieving stress because it is said to play a big role in quieting the sympathetic nervous system, "the fight or flight" response to stress.

To quote a Harvard Medical School newsletter, "When we sense a threat, our fight-or-flight response automatically kicks in. We breathe at a rapid pace to suck in extra oxygen, to fuel our heart and muscles so we can flee the danger.

"Of course, we don't need our fight-or-flight response to escape predators anymore. Our threats now come from the stress of emails, personal confrontations, daily news, and traffic jams."

Stimulation of the vagus nerve can calm over-reactive patterns and positively affect chronic conditions like anxiety and depression. Vagus nerve stimulation can lower heart rate and blood pressure as well. When the vagus nerve is operating optimally, a person can easily switch on the parasympathetic nervous system to shift from a stressed, excited state to a relaxed state. Being able to shift without difficulty to a relaxed state helps to promote good digestion and healthy heart rate variability. Long term, this promotes health for mind and body.

The fastest way to activate the vagus nerve is to immediately modify the quality and tempo of your breathing, as we have been doing throughout the previous exercises when you take deep, full inhalations and release your out-going breath in long, slow exhalations. When you are stressed, breathing is often short and shallow. Conversely, when you are relaxed, breathing is deeper and slower.

In his book, *Accessing the Healing Power of the Vagus Nerve: Self-Help Exercises for Anxiety, Depression, Trauma, and Autism*, Stanley Rosenberg expands on recent, important discoveries about the vagus nerve in the human nervous system. Rosenberg highlights the vital role of the proper functioning of the vagus nerve, and he explores simple ways we can regulate its optimal function to relax deeply, improve sleep, and recover from injury and trauma. If you want to know more about the vagus nerve, I recommend his book.

The next, and last, exercise chapter consists of one simple pose from a prone position, on the belly. All there is to do is to lie on your stomach, turn your head to one side, move your leg into position, and relax! It is truly a great way to end your exercises in bed. Watch out though. You may get so relaxed that you fall back to sleep. Better set your alarm.

Chapter 10

Exercise 10: Relief for Lower Back and Sciatica Pain

Half-Frog Pose

This is a simple pose. Once in position, hold for at least a minute while you relax. If you are comfortable, hold the pose longer. Once you know this pose, you may be able to incorporate it into a sleeping position in the early morning hours of sleep.

This pose helps release tension in your lower back. Half-Frog Pose also relaxes the piriformis muscle, which is sometimes the cause of irritation of the sciatic nerve and can cause pain in your buttock, and often down the back and side of your leg.

- Lie on your stomach without a pillow.
- Turn your head to one side.
- Bend the knee on that side.
- Move that leg up so that the thigh is as much of a right angle to your body as is comfortable. Choose comfort for this pose.

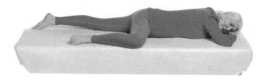

- Hold for 2 minutes or longer if you are comfortable.

If one side or the other causes discomfort, do just the side that feels good.

Keep trying both sides each time you practice. With time, you may be able to do both sides with comfort, if unable to do so in the beginning.

You have made it all the way through the 10 exercises. Congratulations!

Woohoo!

When you are ready to get out of bed, move slowly as you stand up. Pause.

Become aware of the bottoms of your feet with your weight evenly distributed on the inner and outer edges of your feet. Contract your leg muscles to feel long, firm legs rising from your feet to your hips. Feel the lift of your spine all the way to your head.

The previous stretches and movement sequences you have done have helped to realign your upright posture. Can you feel it? This is Standing Mountain Pose.

Notice the effects of the exercises you have completed. What do you perceive? An awakened awareness of your body, from the inside as well as outside? An experience of connection and presence? Add your smile.

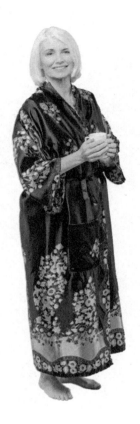

The next chapter is one to use at the end of the day, as you climb into bed and get ready to sleep. Turn the page to see how.

Chapter 11

The Best Rest: Deep Relaxation

1. The Importance of Relaxation
2. Sponge Pose, Called Savasana
3. Aids for Total Comfort
4. Progressive Relaxation/Body Scan
5. Tense and Release Relaxation

"The time to relax is when you don't have time for it."
— Sydney J. Harris

Two Different Approaches to Relaxation

1. Progressive Relaxation
2. Tense the Muscles and Release

Do not skip over this section.

1. The Importance of Relaxation

It is vitally important to learn how to relax, and to be able to relax at will. Your body while asleep is not as relaxed as you can get.

Learn how to relax your body so that, on the subtlest level, your muscles are tension free and your energy flows without blockages. Deep relaxation allows an abundant flow of your life force to all organs, glands, nerves, and cells in your body. With the free flow of your life-force energy, the functioning of your immune system is greatly enhanced.

Being able to relax at will brings greater comfort to muscles that may be habitually tight. Relaxation also brings ease to your mind—a state of calm, well-being in the place of worry or overload. Imagine going through your day feeling focused and at ease.

Being able to relax at will is a tool you can use whenever you feel the need to change a physically or mentally stressed state into a place of greater balance and peace.

Who does not need a resource like that for body and mind in today's stressful world?

And the good news? It is easier to relax than you think. The more you practice, the better you get.

2. Sponge Pose, called *Savasana*

- Begin in a relaxed pose on your back. It may feel most comfortable to have a small pillow under your head and another pillow under your knees or thighs to help your lower back relax and be more comfortable.

Be intentional about the placement of your limbs:

- Separate your legs so they are wider than hip-width.

- Place your arms away from your sides, half-way between your shoulders and hips. Turn your palms up.

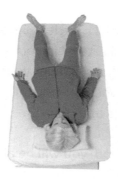

3. Aids for Total Comfort

To create more opening in your chest:

- Press your right elbow into the bed enough to lift your right shoulder and shoulder blade up; then roll your shoulder down and tuck your shoulder blade down to rest it on the bed.
- Do the same on the other side with the left elbow, shoulder, and shoulder blade.

What follows are two different approaches to relaxation. Both will lead to a deeper state of relaxation than just lying down on the bed.

The first method is called a "progressive relaxation." With this approach, you concentrate on relaxing each muscle in every part of the body, from the eyes down to the toes.

Most people who use this approach start with relaxation in the feet and progressively work upwards. I suggest the opposite. Begin with the muscles of your face, specifically your eyes, then cheeks, jaw, and lips.

Why start relaxing your facial muscles? Because your facial muscles take up a large amount of "real estate" in your brain. By quieting your brain, you can more quickly and easily quiet your entire system. Humans are visually oriented beings who use language (thus the need to quiet the brain activity for your eyes and mouth).

When you learn this method, you will be able to relax your entire body. You will decrease tension in your muscles and rest deeply, in a peaceful and restorative state for body and mind.

4. Progressive Relaxation/Body Scan

Begin with your face, and entire head and neck.

- Bring your attention to your eyes. Without moving your head, look upwards toward the ceiling and focus on one spot. Keep your eyes open and look at that one place above you. When the eye muscles feel tired, close your eyelids and bring your awareness to your eyes—the eyes themselves, the eyelids, and the muscles around your eyes.
- Create a sensation of ease and relaxation in the eye area. Take your time. Don't be in a hurry to relax.
- Next, imagine the relaxed sensation you experience in and around your eyes, sliding up into your forehead. Think about the skin of your forehead, and imagine your forehead skin soft and very smooth, with any lines of tension or tiredness just melting away. Keep your attention on your forehead and slowly spread the relaxation in your

forehead all the way across to your temples.

- Move the feeling of comfort down over to your temples and behind your ears. Then...down into your cheeks, and really relax your cheek muscles.
- When the relaxation has built in the cheeks, move that comfortable sensation to your jaw muscles...deep into those jaw muscles...then down farther and over to your chin.
- As the relaxation fills your chin, let that relaxation move up into your lips so that your lips become soft and full and totally relaxed.
- Be aware of this mask of softness, an experience of complete relaxation that you create in all your facial muscles.
- Now imagine or think about drawing the relaxation all the way up to the crown of your head...up to the very top of your head.
- Think about sending this relaxation through all of your scalp muscles. Send the relaxation slowly flowing down the back of your head, all the way down through your neck muscles. Take your time.
- Let your neck muscles absorb the relaxation so that every muscle in your neck softens and relaxes deeply.
- Create complete relaxation through all the muscles in your neck and head and face.

2. The second step is to completely relax your shoulders and send the relaxation through your arms and hands. Imagine comfort overflowing the shoulders and moving that wonderful feeling down into your upper arm area...lower arm...through the wrists...into the hands and out the fingers. Go slowly and take your time, focusing on each part of your arms, joints, and hands.

3. The third step is to send relaxation to your torso... relaxation moving from the shoulders into the front side of the torso, through the muscles of the chest...in and around the stomach...moving the relaxation

through the internal organs and tissues...slowly all the way to your hips. Imagine, as the relaxation flows through your organs, the organs soften, and this causes them to function at peak performance.

4. From your shoulders, send the relaxation into your back, relaxing the upper back muscles, those of your midback, and especially down into the lower back and buttocks. Include all the muscles that run along your spine, from your neck to your tail bone.

5. From your hips, increase the relaxation by sending a feeling of comfort and ease down into your thighs...then in and around your knees...and through your lower legs...past the ankles...and down into your feet all the way to the tips of your toes.

6. Become aware of your total body relaxing...your feet and legs...hands and arms...all of your torso...front and back...and your neck and head.

Rest deeply, experiencing your body as one unit.

During your relaxation, you may become aware of currents of energy throughout your body. Imagine this as the circulation of your life force to every part of your being.

Rest...and renew...and drift off to sleep.

Or, if you desire to return to your waking consciousness:

- Bring your attention to your hands and feet, fingers and toes. Gently begin to move them.
- Stretch your limbs.
- Bend your knees and bring your feet to the bed.

- Pull your knees into your chest.
- Roll over to one side. Take a breath or two before pushing yourself up to a seated position.

5. Tense and Release Relaxation

For some people, tensing or tightening the muscles first, before letting go into relaxation, works better in achieving a deep relaxation. When you increase sensation through tightening the muscles first, you may be able to let go of tension all at once. This method may make your relaxation more palpable and easier to notice.

To clarify, you focus on a part of your body, tighten the muscles in that part, squeezing that part very tight...then quickly release and relax.

Start on the right with the right hand and arm:

- Tighten the muscles of your hand into a fist; make the arm muscles tight...tight, and even tighter, and raise your arm off the surface of the bed...then completely relax.
- Release the muscles; release the tightness. Let your right arm become very loose and comfortable.
- Take a deep breath in and a full breath out.
- Do that again. This time, spread the fingers of your right hand. Open your fingers wide. Tighten the muscles of your hand and your arm, all the way to your shoulder.
- Hold the muscles tight, tighter...now, immediately relax. Release any tension in your right hand and arm.
- Again, take a deep breath in...and out. At the end of each cycle of tightening and release, add this breath. As you exhale, look for any remaining tension in the muscles and let it go with the breath.

Move to the left side:

- Make a fist with your left hand. Tighten the muscles of your hand and fist and arm. Lift the arm off the bed as you do this.
- Squeeze the muscles tight...tighter...all the way...and now release.
- Relax the muscles of your left hand and arm and release your arm to the bed.
- Tighten your hand again. This time, open your fingers wide, spread your fingers...and make the muscles of your fingers, hand and arms tight.
- Tight, tighter...and now release...and relax.

Both hands and arms together:

- Make two fists.
- Squeeze the fists and tighten the muscles of both arms. Lift them up.
- Hold them tight, tighter...and release. Relax your hands and arms.

Repeat with both hands and arms:

- This time, open your hands and spread your fingers wide.
- Engage the muscles in your hands and arms, making all the muscles tight... muscles firm. Tight, tighter...and release.
- Relax completely the muscles of your arms and hands.
- Remember to take your deep breath in...and out.

Keep your arm muscles relaxed and bring the tightening exercise down to each leg and foot, starting on the right:

- Tighten the muscles of your right leg.

- Flex your ankle. Bring your toes up. Press through your heel.
- Make all the muscles in your foot and leg so tight, tight...tighter.
- Now let go and relax.

Repeat, pointing your toes this time.

- Point your toes.
- Firm the muscles of your foot and leg.
- Hold them tight, tighter...then release.
- Relax...

Move to your left leg.

- Tighten the muscles of your left leg.
- Flex your ankle. Bring your toes up. Press through your heel.
- Make all the muscles in your foot and leg so tight, tight...tighter.
- Now let go and relax.

Repeat, pointing your toes.

- Point your toes.
- Firm the muscles of your foot and leg.
- Hold them tight, tighter...then release.
- Relax...

Both legs and feet at the same time:

- Tighten the muscles of both legs. You can even lift your feet and legs off the floor.
- Flex your ankles. Bring your toes up. Press through your heels.
- Make all the muscles in your feet and legs so tight, tight...tighter.

- Now let go and release.

Repeat, pointing your toes.

- Point your toes.
- Firm the muscles of your feet and legs.
- Hold them tight, tighter...then release.
- Relax...all the muscles of the legs and feet, very relaxed.

Become aware of your arms, hands, feet, and legs, now completely relaxed.

All four limbs at the same time:

- Making fists and tightening the muscles of the hands and arms, feet and legs also tight, tight...tighter, and release. Deep breath in...and out.
- Take a moment to sense that relaxation in the limbs.

Do that again, and this time add all of the muscles of your torso, your belly, chest, and all of your back.

- Tighten your feet, your legs, your hips, and the muscles of your belly, chest, and back, and your shoulders, arms, and hands.
- Make all the muscles very tight...and release.
- Soften all the muscles...relax all the muscles.
- Take a deep breath in...and out.

Keep the muscles of the body relaxed and move to the muscles of your face as you take a deep breath in:

- Tighten only the muscles of your forehead. Frown, scowl, and scrunch up your forehead muscles.
- Add the eye muscles and squeeze your eyes tight.
- Add your cheeks and jaw muscles and your lips and squeeze all those muscles.
- As you breathe out, relax all your facial muscles.
- Do the face tightening once again and add all the muscles of your body, tensing your whole body as you breathe in.
- Breathe out and relax all your muscles...every muscle becoming loose and totally relaxed.
- With each following exhalation for the next several breaths, imagine letting all your muscles let go even more.
- Stay with this relaxation at least five minutes to allow your body and mind to appreciate the benefits of a total relaxation.

Chapter 12

Adding a Habit

1. Tiny Habits
2. What Do You Want?
3. Choosing Your Response
4. From Ziplining to Swimming to You

> *"A year from now, you'll be glad you started today."*
> — Karen Lamb

Yoga has become popular in the U.S. in recent years due to its benefits to overall well-being, health, and peace of mind. Yoga is ubiquitous; classes have sprung up everywhere. That was until the pandemic, COVID-19, when most of us had to limit our exposure to groups and gatherings.

I continue to teach weekly through live, online classes. In my classes, I present poses and breathing techniques that I hope will stay with my students beyond that class, and maybe get incorporated into a student's daily activity, doing yoga every day.

That is what happened to a student named Cherie.

As you try the 10 exercises, know that you will benefit from each in a different way. Every exercise is also complete. You will likely feel both immediate and, over time, long-term effects, like Cherie.

There are many benefits to daily/weekly stretching, strengthening, and relaxation exercises. When you have a comprehensive program, you aid every system in the body. You feel better all over and are calmer and more focused for the day ahead.

1. Tiny Habits

Because the 10 exercise chapters can be practiced one at a time, you see that you can take your practice in bite-sized portions. Try several of the exercises each day, first thing after you are awake. Over time, the stretches may become a daily habit.

Dr. B. J. Fogg is a research scientist at Stanford University. His mission is helping people form new habits. He recommends breaking any desired activity into very small, actionable steps, and creating a "tiny habit." In Fogg's book, *Tiny Habits: The Small Changes That Change Everything* (2020), he says to break desired goals down into small, simple steps. Start with a tiny habit to create big change. Tiny habits are easy to do and help us stay motivated to stick with the new behavior or activity long term.

That is why I recommend starting with Exercise 1 and doing that exercise sequence every day. Those simple foot and ankle stretches will reinforce doing exercise in bed. After doing Exercise 1, you might want to put together a short program each day to explore what the exercises can do. For example, doing Exercises 2 and 3 may feel quite good for your hips. Exercises 4 and 5 will work wonders for your back, and Exercise 6 will benefit both hips and back. Exercises 7 and 8 stretch your thighs—inner, outer, back, and front—and lubricate your hip joints as well. Exercises 9 and 10 function as specific remedies.

You will find the exercises that work best for you. On the days when you have more time, you may want to do them all.

2. What Do You Want?

This brings up a bigger question about taking care of yourself, your whole being.

One of the most important questions you can ask yourself—about everything—is, "What do you want?" Ask it of yourself concerning your body's strength, flexibility, mobility, or overall vitality. Ask that question to find out how you want to feel and how you want your mind to function. "What do you want?" is a powerful inquiry. It is valid to ask it even if what you really want does not seem possible.

On the other hand, what if you are unclear about what you want? In that case, it may be easier to think of what you do not want (e.g., my back hurting all the time), and change the "not wanting" to what you do want instead.

Here is a suggestion for a written exercise: Draw a line down the middle of the page and label the two columns: "Don't Want" and "Do Want." Start with "Don't Want" and come up with a list. Next to each "Don't Want," write a "Do Want." For example, if "I don't want to feel so tired all the time" is on your "Don't Want" list, put "I want to feel energized and well" on the "Do Want" side. Change "I don't want back pain!" to "I want my back to feel great and pain-free!"

Once you know what you want, draw a line through the "Don't Want" item and say out loud, "I choose to _____," and fill in the blank with what you do want.

This has been a powerful exercise for me and has helped me create a life that I truly love in all areas. What you want can be physical or material, emotional or spiritual, and may have to do with your health, happiness, and success in your chosen endeavors.

3. Choosing Your Response

Sometimes a solution lies in changing the way you think about a problem. A change in attitude can shift the way you perceive an event or activity. I had an unexpected breakthrough when I became aware of what I did not want and focused on what I did want; in particular, how I wanted to feel.

4. From Ziplining to Swimming to You

While attending a conference in Costa Rica, I had an opportunity to try ziplining through a rain forest. The idea of that kind of adventure sounded exciting. But as I thought about it, I began to doubt whether I would enjoy the rush of adrenaline I was bound to experience; I was afraid.

Many of my friends signed up for the excursion and they encouraged me to come with them. "It will be so much fun!"

I said, "OK."

We were transported to the facilities of an outdoor recreation company that offered thrill-seekers the opportunity to "zip" through the forest, while attached by a harness with a pulley, to a cable suspended above the contour of the mountain. The incline was steep; that meant each ride was fast due to gravity's strong pull.

This company was famous for its 12 stations of linked cables that stretched from platform to platform around huge rainforest trees. The 11th cable in the series was purported to be "the longest zipline cable" in the world.

After getting into our harnesses and being checked for safety, we were taken by jeep to the first cable. When we lined up, I went to the rear of the line. I watched in amazement as, one by one, my friends each stepped off the tree platform into thin air and whizzed downward to the next station. I could hear many let out joyful yelps of glee during their rapid descents.

All too soon, it was my turn. I was really scared. But then I just stepped off the platform and whooshed downward. I squeezed my eyes shut. I forgot to breathe! The ride was over quicker than I imagined it would be. There was no time to think much about it as I was unclipped from one cable and attached to another. Each time, I stepped off the platform into nothingness and another fast ride. Each time, I was anxious and afraid. But I got through all 12 cable rides.

I felt pleased that I had conquered my fear enough to complete the entire course. But I did not enjoy the event like others around me seemed to. I thought about how my anxiety and apprehension got in the way of my delight in this unique opportunity. The more I thought about it, the more I wished I could do the whole adventure over, ziplining with confidence rather than fear. After all, I did not come to any harm, so why hold on to the fear?

It was just my luck that on the day the conference ended, there was a massive snowstorm on the east coast of the U.S. where I live. Most of the conference attendees were returning to the west coast and were unaffected by the snowstorm. But most flights to the east coast were cancelled, mine included. I found myself with an extra day at the resort. In the morning, I met two remaining friends at breakfast and the three of us came up with a plan for our free day. You might guess what we chose: ziplining!

I liked the idea of having a second chance to create a different outcome. I wanted to lean into the ride instead of holding back with hesitation. I asked myself, why not just have fun this time with no worry? I created a clear picture in my imagination: stepping off the tree platform with abandon and being thrilled by the ride. The positive mental image excited me about the opportunity for a "do-over."

That decision was powerful. During this second chance, I approached each step off the tree platforms without reluctance and with an expectation of fun. What a difference the shift in attitude made. I remembered to take good, long breaths, and I got great enjoyment from my altered approach! We three had so much fun that day. That ziplining adventure turned out to be one of the peak experiences of my life.

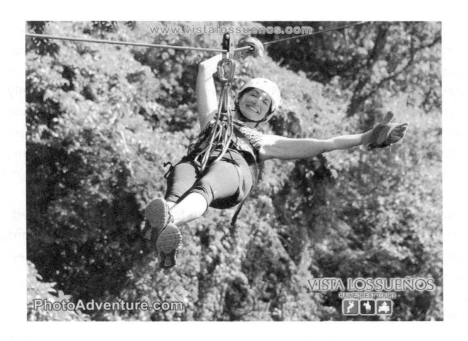

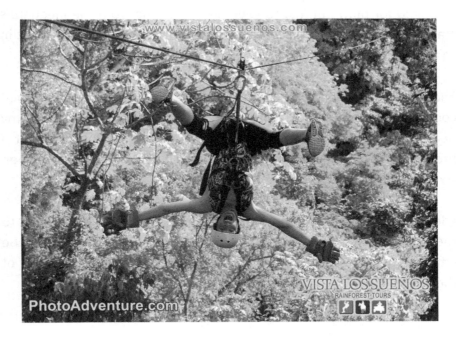

This story of transformation did not stop there. I live in New Hampshire, near beautiful Dublin Lake, a 200+ acre body of water at the foot of Mount Monadnock. (It is the mountain that holds the distinction of being the most climbed mountain in the world; I think because it is only 3,145 feet high.) The lake stretches nearly a mile long and a half mile wide and is 100 feet deep. The water is so cold that most swimmers venture in only during the months of July and August, when the water is as warm as it gets.

2020 was the summer of COVID-19 and our little beach club was closed. No dock or rafts were put out into the water, and there was no lifeguard on duty. It was "swim at your own risk." That kept many swimmers away. It was ideal for me.

Most often, I went for a refreshing immersion at the end of the workday before dinner. My husband went with me to the lake, not into the water (too cold for him) but just to keep an eye on me from the lifeguard's stand. I did appreciate his company and him being there for me just in case I had trouble.

Though I had learned how to swim when a child, I had never developed confidence as a swimmer. Whenever I got into water that was over my head, I would begin to think about drowning. That fear was not a problem if swimming in a swimming pool, but it always arose when swimming in the lake.

I do not like being limited by fear. I set a goal for myself to swim out to the farthest buoy, the spot where a floating raft would normally be attached to a cable deep below. It represented the outer boundary of the beach club.

Luckily, one day, the beach club's swimming teacher showed up to swim when I was there. We started talking and I asked her if she could give me swimming lessons to make my stroke and form better. She said no, not this summer, but then she watched me swim and gave me a few tips. I decided to become a stronger swimmer despite my fear of being in water over my head.

My desire, determination, and commitment to overcome my anxiety about the water now felt exhilarating, like how I felt on my "do-over" experience ziplining. If I could change my approach in the trees, could I change my experience in the water?

Yes! But change did not happen in one session like it had happened with ziplining. I had to practice and increase my abilities day by day, just like I am asking you to do with these yoga stretches from bed.

Swimming is now my new summer passion. Now, when I am in the lake water, I feel like I am swimming in liquid silk. It gives me so much pleasure; a pleasure that I unknowingly deprived myself of for years and years.

What is waiting for you?

I recommend that you move your body every day. Move your bones, your muscles, and the connective tissue that holds the inside of your body together. Adding a few daily stretches and yoga poses, before you even get out of bed for the day, may open a new door for you. How would it be to move towards more resilience and ease, and to a greater love and care for your body?

I continue to seek resilience. I am still learning and adapting yoga and movement to my body even after more than 50 years of practice. New health habits and new ways to think and move may be our best preventative medicine—a prescription for a happy and healthy life. I wish that for you.

Final Words of Inspiration

There are so many things in life that are hard.
This is not one of them.

Doing the exercises once does not
make the imbalance go away forever.

Your body needs daily attention.
It is the price you pay for generating ease.

Do not worry if you are doing it perfectly.
Just start and pay attention.

When we are informed, we make better choices.

Nothing changes nothing;
doing something may change everything.

It is time for extreme self-care.

About the Author

Peggy Cappy is the creator of *Yoga for the Rest of Us*, a popular PBS series about yoga that has raised millions of dollars for public television over the past 20 years. Peggy has created program after program exploring the different benefits of yoga practice. Her yoga is based on the premise that everyone, regardless of age or ability, can benefit from yoga, meditation, and breathing techniques.

Peggy's unique, adaptive approach to yoga has adults finding they have energy, flexibility, and peace of mind they never dreamed possible. She shares her passion for yoga and meditation through workshops and classes, teacher training, presentations and special events, videos, books, and CDs. www.PeggyCappy.com

Peggy Cappy has traveled the world as an anthropologist, living for two years with an indigenous tribe in Papua New Guinea more than 50 years ago, supported by National Geographic, through which she made a documentary film with her husband. She has spent months in India in ashrams, has meditated in the mountain caves where the sage Ramana Maharshi lived, and felt the power of meditating alone in the Great Pyramid in Egypt.

Peggy holds a B.A. degree in dance, a B.A. in anthropology, a PH.D. in medical hypnotherapy, and has scores of advanced certifications in yoga and meditation. Her previous books include *Yoga for All of Us* (St. Martin's Press), and *My Father's Stories: Experiences of a Prisoner of War in World War II*.

Peggy is grateful for her membership in the Transformational Leadership Council, a group of world leaders committed to making the world a better place. It was founded by Jack Canfield, co-author of the *Chicken Soup for the Soul* series and the *Success Principles*.

A mother of a grown daughter and son, Peggy is a grandmother to four. She is nourished by time in nature, kayaking, swimming, and hiking in the beautiful wilds surrounding her home in New Hampshire at the foot of Mt. Monadnock, America's most hiked mountain.

Made in the USA
Coppell, TX
24 November 2024

40581633R00066